THE MONK

THE MONK

BRETT GARAMELLA

iUniverse, Inc.
New York Lincoln Shanghai

THE MONK

iUniverse books may be ordered through booksellers or by contacting:

iUniverse
2021 Pine Lake Road, Suite 100
Lincoln, NE 68512
www.iuniverse.com
1-800-Authors (1-800-288-4677)

ISBN-13: 978-0-595-38626-0 (pbk)
ISBN-13: 978-0-595-83006-0 (ebk)
ISBN-10: 0-595-38626-1 (pbk)
ISBN-10: 0-595-83006-4 (ebk)

Printed in the United States of America

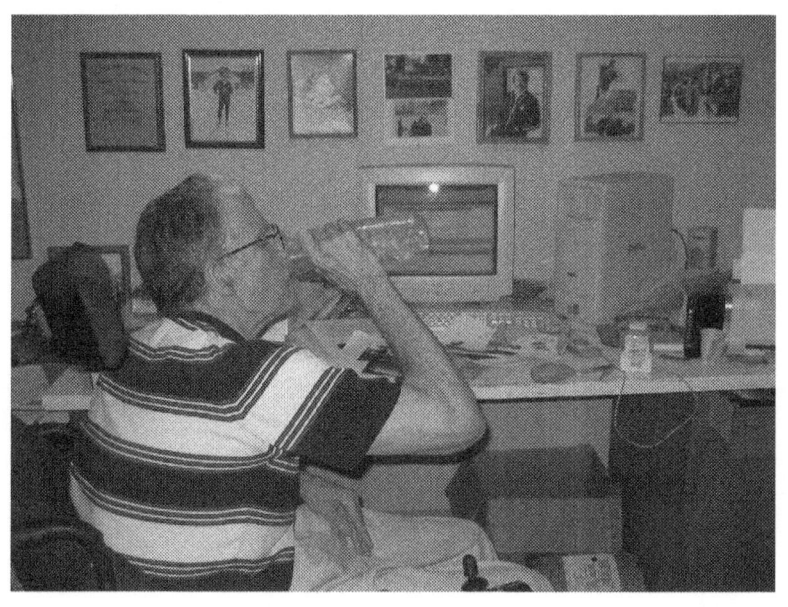

He's just a well-rounded individual, and he had so much going for him. So he was a big inspiration for all of us.... we loved him.

—Chris Nice, doctor living in Hanover, N.H.

He's still a remarkable person. He does so many things that nobody else in his position could possibly do.

—Steve Daniels, head judge, Government Services Board of Contract Appeals, living in Washington, D.C.

To meet him, to sit with him for an hour, is to be in awe. Just awe.

—Carroll Brewster, retired, former Dartmouth College dean living in Ridgefield, Conn.

Monk is a true hero in my book right now. It's sort of easy to say this. You look back and you idealize a person or you idealize something. But I would say that Monk was a hero of mine before this happened.

—Marshall "Buzz" Land, pediatrician living in Shelburne, Vt.

Above his cluttered desk, where he sits by most of the time now, there are six framed photographs and a plaque hanging in a row on the wall. They are his "cream of the crop." Sometimes when he looks at them it is as if he were there again, competing with the best in the world and traveling to places a kid from his hometown could only imagine by looking at a magazine picture. Back then, he never knew how much those photos would mean to him later in life. He never knew he would need them to keep his sanity. How could he? He was in ski heaven, playing with the Gods. It was the perfect place for him at that time in his life. No problem moving his legs. No problem cracking jokes with his buddies. No problem, despite shyness, talking to a young, pretty woman. And no idea of what lay ahead for him. Nope, those photos were taken before his life began to unravel....

This is a cross-country skier story. But, more importantly, it is a story about life and how to make the most of it no matter what hand you're dealt. Monk has seen some of the best and worst hands, and played them both. A lot of his life today has to do with his past, even if that past appears in spontaneous flashbacks. Quite ironic for a man who has always looked ahead. To help us understand why a 59-year-old man still smiles and laughs as if he isn't sitting in a wheelchair in an old-age home, we must first, however, go back to those photos.

Take a look at the third one from the left. That's Monk as a 14 year old. See how he's soaring over a ridge with his knees tucked in the air and the Matterhorn taking up half the picture in the background. It's one of his best childhood memories. Monk's father, Lyman "Perry" Williams, took that black and white photo of him in the spring of 1961. At the time, trips to Europe were still a novelty. It was the first time Monk had left the United States. He had gone with Perry, his mother Ruth Kelley, and other Snow Ridge skiers. Snow Ridge was the small ski area back home that his parents ran. At age 3 or 4, Monk began skiing. From their home in Boonville, N.Y., his parents drove 10 miles north to Snow Ridge, located in the tiny town of Turin. They always brought Monk with them. "Cheap babysitters," he says of the many other Snow Ridge skiers then. So before he knew any better skiing was the biggest part of his life. But there really wasn't much else to do in rural upstate New York. Monk would later joke with his college and ski friends about being from Boonville, because it sounds like "boondocks." There were just over two-thousand residents and one traffic light in town. When he talks about his childhood stories now, he refers to them as "Boonville bullshit," which makes some sense considering it was a small farming town with lots of cows and manure. However, he has vivid memories of building snow tunnels from his house on Main Street to the house of his best friend David Harvey, who lived next door. Monk still has a postcard of a snowmobile race in his hometown; however, he never attended the race because he was always skiing. On the back of the postcard it reads: "Boonville is the Snowmobile Capital of the World…Snowfall winter 1972 over 309 inches."

Monk lived in a traditional household of his generation. Perry had the final say in any decision, and Ruth was the one Monk and his older brother, Dick, could talk to if they had a problem. More often than not, it was easier to talk to her since Perry was a full-time lawyer and spent his free time year-round at Snow Ridge. By the time Monk was born on July 2, 1946, Perry and Ruth were much more involved in the ski area than when Dick was a child. In fact, Snow Ridge didn't exist then. When Ruth was pregnant with Monk in the fall of 1945, she and Perry trekked up and down a hill just north of Boonville to lay out the slopes that became Snow Ridge. The eight-year difference in age made Dick and Monk feel more like an uncle and nephew than brothers. Although not really close to one another because of the age difference, they both enjoyed similar activities. When they weren't on the ski slopes, they hiked and camped and canoed as Boy Scouts in the Adirondacks. To the right of his desk there is a photo on the wall of Perry shaking Monk's hand for becoming an Eagle Scout at age 13. Though Monk loved all the outdoor activities as a Scout, he didn't have much choice. In 1928 Perry had become the first Eagle Scout in Lewis and Jefferson County; therefore his son would do the same.

Neither of the boys was born with exceptional hand-eye coordination nor athletic ability. Monk tried baseball and basketball but his eyes didn't focus together so he had a problem with depth perception. Instead, he loved hiking up the Adirondack high-peaks, such as Blue Mountain, the same mountain his parents had spent their 1931 honeymoon after meeting at the University at Albany. Little did he know hiking was great preparation for his near future.

As a freshman at Boonville Central High School in 1960, Monk was a three-event skier. One of the events was cross-country, which he thought he'd try for the first time. By his account he wasn't very good on the used, wooden skis the coach had let him borrow. In his mind he had aspirations of becoming a great alpine skier like his brother, who had just finished his college career at St. Lawrence University. He didn't want to be another "hick" from a town that was more known for farming than skiing. And growing up, his shy demeanor around girls hurt his love life. Skiing at an elite level would prove he was "a stud." After seeing Renie Cox and Ken Phelps compete at the 1960 Olympics as members of the U.S. Ski Team, Monk dreamed of making the Olympics as an alpine skier. Cox and Phelps had both skied at Snow Ridge growing up and Monk knew Phelps's father. On the other hand, his talents seemed more suited for cross-country. Three times in high school he suffered concussions after crashing into a tree while alpine skiing and wearing an old leather helmet with rubber lining like those worn by WWII pilots.

One weekend in January 1962, Monk and his ski teammates, who called themselves the Ski Bums, raced against Deerfield Academy in Massachusetts. With hopes of skiing stardom, he had an informal interview with the Deerfield staff. Monk saw it as an opportunity to meet classmates who didn't have a farming background. Besides, Boonville didn't have a pool and hockey rink and big basketball gym like Deerfield had. When he returned and told his parents he wanted to enroll at Deerfield, they were pleased.

At Deerfield Academy Monk earned his nickname. In Boonville, people called him by his birth name, Steve Williams. Each morning at Deerfield, he sliced bananas into his cereal. His buddies called him "Monkey" for about a week and then it was shortened to "Monk." The nickname continued to follow him and he liked it better than Steve.

It sometimes suited him well on the ski slope, where he monkeyed around. One day his junior year he tried to jump over a snowdrift on a bridge at the bottom of Snow Ridge. He crashed and injured his right knee. Although he returned to the slopes two weeks later, his knee had cartilage and ligament problems the rest of his career.

When deciding on life after Deerfield, Monk applied to Brown, Dartmouth and Stanford. His A- average in high school made him a good candidate academically. As a skier, no college recruited him. Of the 155 students in his Deerfield senior class, 11 went to Dartmouth. Monk was one of them.

During his Dartmouth interview, Monk said he used his "best bullshit." As he says holding his nose, "It stunk." He chose Dartmouth for its academic reputation, but more so for its skiing prowess. Deerfield ski coach "Fat Art" Ruggles had graduated from Dartmouth and knew its current cross-country ski coach Al Merrill. Other great Dartmouth skiers had started their ski careers at Deerfield Academy, an easy selling point for ambitious skiers like Monk.

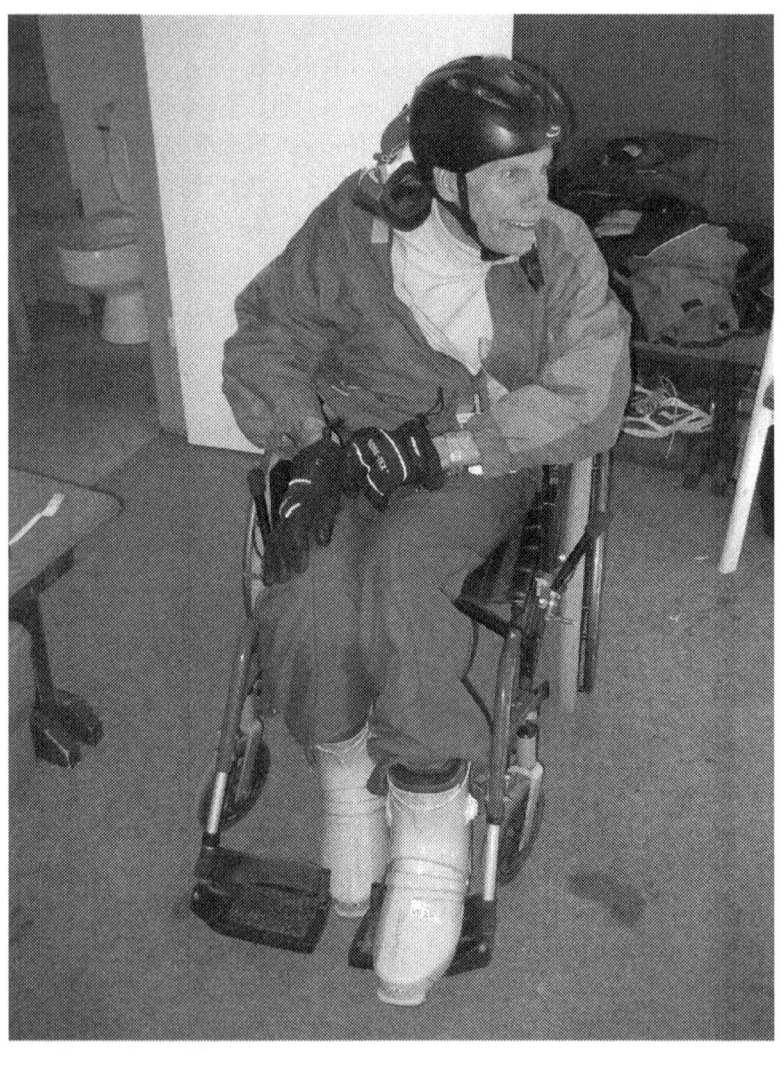

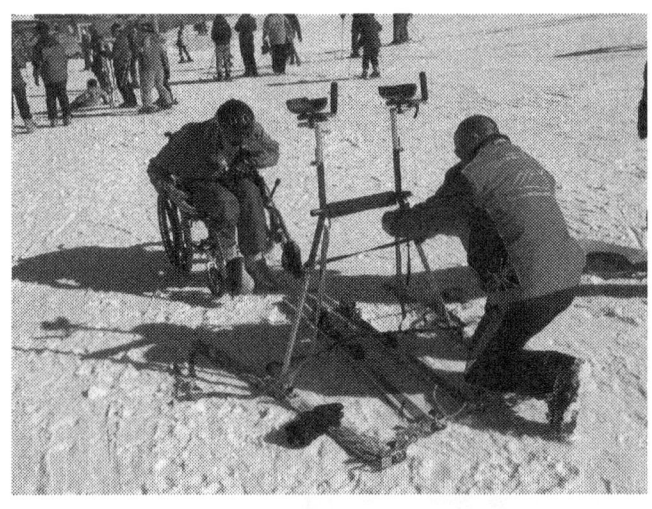

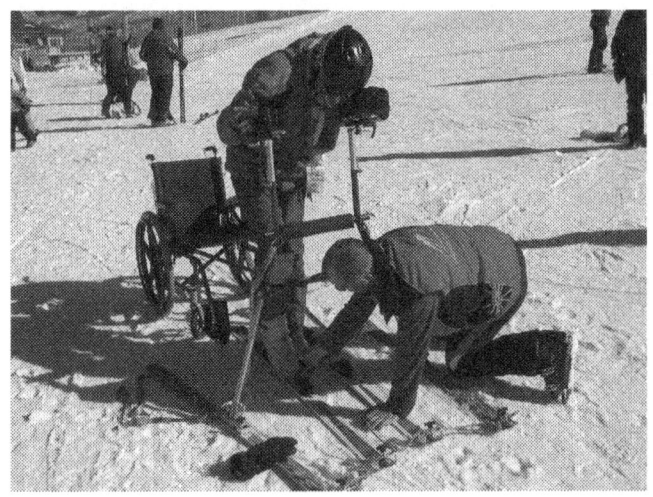

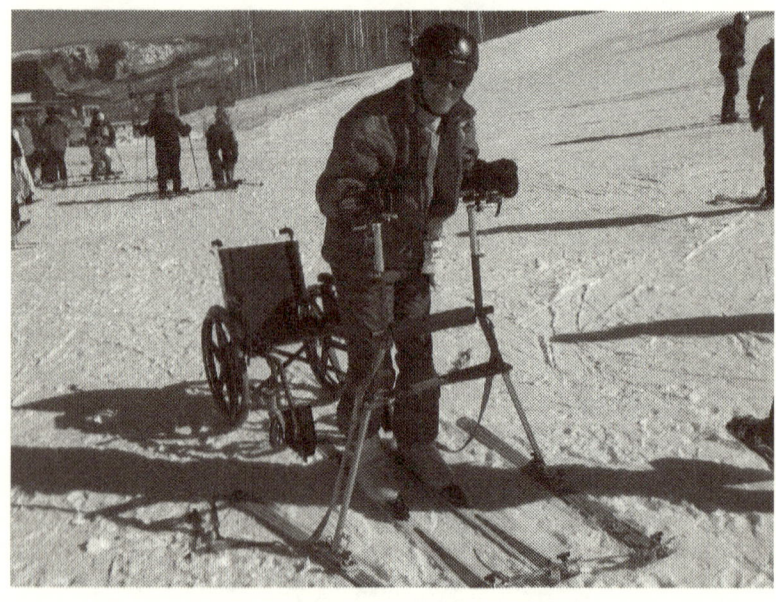

It's human nature to want to be the best at something. For Monk, it became cross-country skiing at Dartmouth. But he didn't tell anyone. He set out to prove to himself and others that he was "a stud." There were no girls to impress at Dartmouth in the 1960s. It wasn't until 1972 that female students were first admitted. So Monk and his buddies went on road trips to Smith College and Wellesley College, two all-girl schools in Massachusetts. When asked what his college friends would do if they met a girl they liked and wanted to hook up, he said with a smile, "Hit and run." He had more time his freshman year to go on road trips; because of a bum right knee, Monk did not ski that year. However, he wanted to be a part of the cross-country ski team so Merrill made him manager.

Merrill was the Dartmouth head ski coach and head U.S. Nordic Ski Team coach from 1956 to 1970. His Dartmouth teams never finished lower than fourth nationally. The "Silver Fox's" dedication and love of the sport rubbed off on Monk. Silver Fox, they gave Merrill that nickname because of his silver-colored hair and unmatched knowledge on waxing skis. Before races other teams tried spying on him, which was the norm in those days, for a glimpse of the particular wax he had in his hands. Merrill and other coaches switched waxing containers; they might put a red wax in a green tin. He knew more than waxing skis. He was one of the first coaches to use calisthenics with mini trampolines, and implemented other innovative exercises such as hill running with poles. His training was so advanced that none of his skiers ran for the Dartmouth cross-country team in the fall because they knew Merrill's demanding workouts would help them more.

Because of Merrill, Monk's Olympic dream changed from alpine to cross-country skiing. That change occurred in March of Monk's freshman year when he bonded with Merrill for the first time on a trip from Hanover, N.H., to Stowe, Vt., for the Sugar Slalom race. (After the race the skiers poured sugar on snow and ate it, a New England treat). Monk admired Merrill's ski knowledge and likeable personality, in particular his "great belly laugh" as they rode to Stowe in his Chevy Nova.

By that summer Monk's knee had healed, but his injury list wasn't complete. He loved to waterski. He impressed his friends going barefoot and standing on his slalom ski. He may have felt invincible at the time, but he crashed while waterskiing at the Fourth Lake in the Fulton Chain of Lakes in upstate New York. He dislocated his left shoulder, an injury that prevented him from going to the Vietnam War.

In the fall of 1966, Monk joined Psi Upsilon, a fraternity to which many Dartmouth skiers pledged in those days. Although Monk loved fraternity life, he had other interests.

"Monk was as much fun as anybody, but he was also one of the hardest working guys I ever met," says Marshall "Buzz" Land, a fraternity brother who was a year ahead of Monk. "Everybody would be coming back from studying and Monk would still be working."

Monk's strong work ethic helped him become a Rufus Choate Scholar, the highest yearly honor at Dartmouth. Studying, however, wasn't his top priority, and to his peers he was always one of the guys. Good times and memorable moments were as common as his big smile and contagious laugh.

"I will say that the fraternity I was in, I would say that I've never seen a group of people that had more infectious smiles," says Land. "And number one is the Monk."

His friends saw Monk, an economics major, studying with headphones on. Monk loved listening to rock n' roll. His favorite song was "Peggy Sue." In addition to studying, he liked listening to the rock n' roll rhythm while lifting weights.

Training, like studying, was not taken lightly. His hard work helped him to earn a spot on Merrill's team as a sophomore, but he did not start. The following summer, in 1966, Monk stayed at his Dartmouth friend and roommate Robbie Peacock's house in Kailua-Kona, a small town on the largest Hawaiian Island, along with another Dartmouth friend, Ned Gillette. Monk and Gillette trained rigorously together, hiking up mountains and volcanos as well as doing running workouts. In midsummer Monk dislocated his shoulder body surfing and returned home. The training paid off. Monk became a starter on the ski team, and Gillette, Monk's cross-country teammate, was the best collegiate skier in the nation that year. Because of Monk's superior physical conditioning, the Dartmouth medical school used him and his slender 6'3" frame in a class as a physical "specimen," putting him through various tests.

His love for skiing—the entire ambiance of it—grew each competitive year. As a Dartmouth senior he was No. 2 on the cross-country team, and that March he won the Eastern Amateur Ski Association 30-kilometer Championships. Skiing helped him meet lifelong friends. He had developed a close relationship with another senior cross-country skier named John Morton, from Middlebury College. The two competed against each other for three years and in their final collegiate race at the NCAA championships in Steamboat Springs, Colo., Morton finished ahead of Monk and second nationally. After the races, they didn't want to head back to the East for classes. Not with all the great snow out West. Besides, they both had a week before spring break. So Monk and Morton and two other Middlebury cross-country skiers talked themselves into skipping classes and spending the next two weeks alpine skiing at Alpine Meadows, Calif., where they joined Bobo Sheehan, who had recently retired as Middlebury ski coach. Since Sheehan managed Alpine Meadows, the ski resort, he set them up in a condominium and gave them lift tickets.

Life couldn't be much better. Another photo. Monk has a picture of the five of them on the lower of the three shelves above his dry bar.

But Monk's skiing career would soon come to a halt. Remember, he never seemed to do anything halfway. In May of his senior year, his fraternity played the Beta house for the interfraternity soccer championship. On one play Monk scored a goal when Beta goalie Gordon Rule, who played football for the Green Bay Packers after graduation, pounced on Monk's right leg. Monk saw a knob sticking out of his knee. Monk, of course, would make the most of this. There is a photo on his shelf of him in his black graduation gown and hat, smiling with crutches and a cast from his waist to ankle.

He fondly remembers having more attention from girls because of his injury.

With his skiing dreams on hold, Monk was admitted into Yale and Harvard law schools. He decided to drive south to New Haven, Conn., for his next year of studies because Yale agreed to accommodate his skiing ambitions. Although skiing took much higher precedence over school, Monk always strove to be the best at everything. Dick says Monk's drive and determination probably came from Perry, who thought being the best was his only option. "By the time he went to law school I was just blown away at how he could get admitted, get these great grades, and to me not look like he was working very hard," Dick says. "And I was always in awe of how much he was learning and how in the mist of all that he was able to ski and have such a great time."

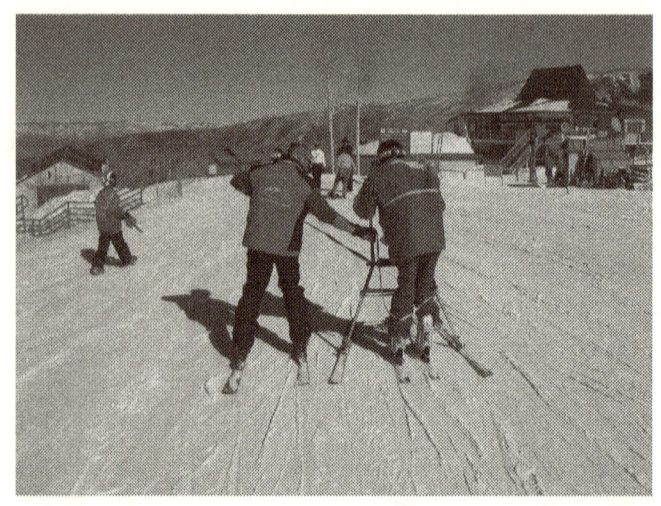

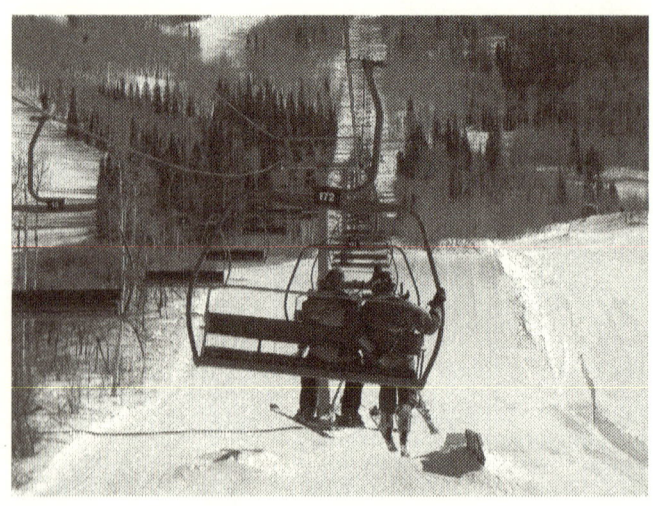

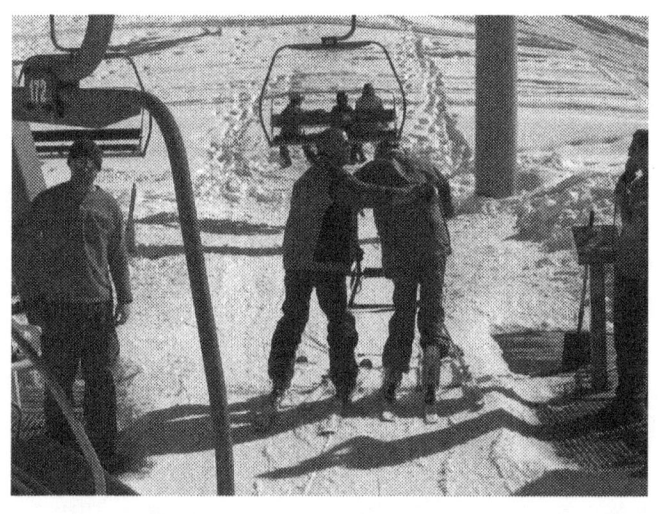

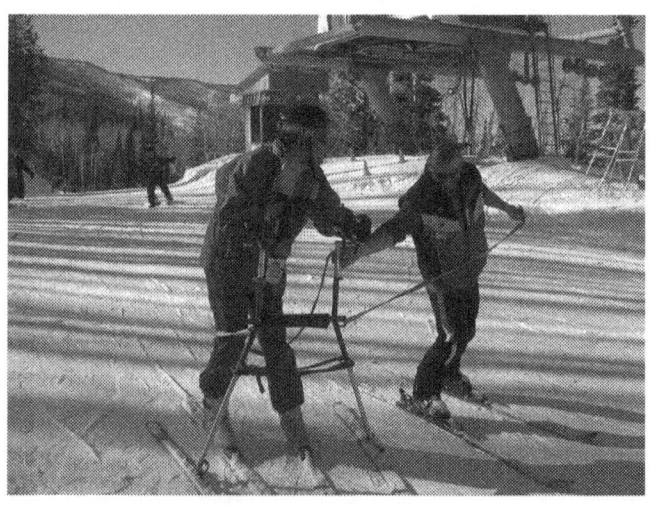

I arrived at Yale in the fall of 1968, the height [or depth] of the "Age of Aquarius," to find most of my peers just hippy, dippy, pot snorters faking being students [or as I affectionately called 'em: "piss ants"], and I was just so disgusted with this sampling of America's brightest and finest minds, I wanted out, loving the pursuit of excellence I saw with Al and his skiers.

Since he had recovered by the fall, Monk attended each U.S. and Eastern cross-country team training camp. Back at Yale he sailed through his classes with his quick wit. His thoughts were more about skiing and the one-quarter Cherokee Indian woman from Connecticut College he had a crush on. He had more success with the skis than with the girl.

His second year at Yale he lived in Madison, Conn., a short drive on Interstate 95 to New Haven. In the middle of January students took their first-term exams. Monk's first test, tax law, was scheduled eight days into the exam period. Following Christmas break, students returned for a two-week reading period. Not Monk. He trained with the U.S. Eastern cross-country team in New Hampshire. No one had seen him at Yale for at least five weeks. So he drove from Madison for his first exam and parked behind the Grove Street Cemetery, where he often did interval training between gravestones. Monk was walking next to the cemetery wall when he spotted an empty whiskey bottle. He grabbed it and continued walking with his books in his other hand. He entered the exam room and sat at his assigned seat at a long wooden table and put his books down. Noticing how nervous and stressed out his classmates looked, Monk slammed the whiskey bottle on the table and *sat back with a big shit-eating grin, trying to look a bit drunk which only confirmed the suspicions of many about my indifference to law school.... when others figured out the bottle was empty, they never forgave me for breaking the mood of their pre-exam tension or nervousness.* The Monkey.

After his second year at Yale, he knew the combination of attending law school and training with the national team was too much. He knew the only way to make the Olympics as a cross-country skier was to take a leave of absence from school, which is what he did for the next two years. Skiing, however, was not the reason for his leave of absence. Carroll Brewster was.

During his first year at Yale, Monk had met Brewster. Brewster had returned to his alma mater (he had graduated from Yale and Yale Law School) to streamline and update the judiciary system in the Sudan. Monk approached Brewster about a job twice the following year since they had become friendly and Brewster had become the dean of students at Dartmouth. Monk wanted a respite from his fellow Yale "piss ants." That summer, in 1970, Monk was working for a law firm in Seattle when Brewster called him, offering Monk a job as his assistant at Dartmouth. Monk gladly obliged.

Monk's dedication to skiing never diminished, even if being an assistant dean caused him to finagle his way out on the crisp cross-country tracks around Hanover. Sometimes in the afternoon, he'd walk by Kay Brock, a well-known Dartmouth secretary of the time, with his skis and she'd say, "Steve, where are you going?"

"I'm going to make a few house calls," he said, and she laughed, and he left and trained.

Skiing consumed his life. For a man who grew up without any idols, skiers such as Bob Gray, Bill Elliott and Mike Gallagher became a source of inspiration. Monk also looked up to Eric "Hammer" Evans, who was the nation's best kayaker from 1970 to 1980. Evans grew up in Hanover, and he skied on the Dartmouth cross-country team, training his enormous upper body in the winter for white-water kayaking. Marty Hall, Eastern Ski Association Nordic program director and later national Nordic team head coach, was friends with Evans and invited him to the national training camp to demonstrate his world-class worth ethic. Monk remembers those training sessions, and one of his favorite ski stories involves how Evans earned his nickname "Hammer." One night during the Christmas holiday in 1970, Monk and some of the best Eastern skiers and Evans gathered at dinner where they were training at Lake Placid, and ate that night at the lodge they roomed. The skiers talked about the new craze in competitive endurance training, which involved maximizing blood sugar to the body's cells. For 20 minutes or so everyone at the table piped into the conversation and tried adding what they knew about science and exercise. Finally, Evans said, "Fuck this blood sugar shit. When you get tired you just put your head down and you hammer." From that point through his competitive career, he was known as the Hammer. "Hammering" away has been Monk's axiom, even long after his days of competitive cross-country skiing.

While not a great technical skier, Monk's effort was rare, even among elite cross-country skiers. One time he trained so hard on a hot summer day at Oak Hill, the local Dartmouth mountain, that medics drove him to the emergency room because of heat exhaustion.

His hard work paid off. In his second year away from Yale, Monk lived with Carroll Brewster and his wife in Hanover. He trained full time, often with his old coach Merrill and other skiers for the 1972 Olympics. When he woke up each morning, he checked his pulse. When he was in his best shape, his resting heart rate beat 35 times per minute. And as usual, he impressed his peers with his drive. Merrill used a trail around Hanover Country Club on the Dartmouth campus, which started and ended on the 18th hole. It was known as "The 10-minute loop" because a good collegiate cross-country runner could finish the hilly course, a total of two miles or so, in 10 minutes. Merrill had the skiers run around the loop three times with a two-minute rest between intervals. One day in the fall of 1971 Monk amazed the others by running the 10-minute loop in about 8:20, setting an unofficial record that was never broken.

He carried that same intensity during his travels at home and abroad.

See the two colored photos in the frame to the right of the Matterhorn picture? They both were taken in Oslo at the Norwegian Ski Games. Look at the bottom photo. A teacher of Monk's from Deerfield Academy, who happened to be there, shot that picture of Monk before the race in early March 1971. What happened in that photo, which was taken before the race, is more important than the actual race. It's snowing out and Monk is signing autographs for a group of Norwegian children with his right hand and holding his freshly waxed skis with his other. It was the first and only time he ever signed autographs and thought to himself, "Why is it *so* good over here?"

Now look at the photo above it. Monk shot that picture two years later, when he and the U.S. Team had just returned to Norway on a sunny day. The Oslo race committee had three red cars they provided to visiting teams. The red station wagon given to the U.S. Team says: "REKORD '73 I HOL-MENKOLLEN" on the left side. On the car's roof is a big red bag filled with the team's skis and poles. A gray Samsonite suitcase with a white U.S. Ski Team logo is showing through the back window. "Suitcase, bag and car," says Monk. "I had to take that picture."

Now take a good look at the black and white photo to the left of the Matterhorn picture. Monk doesn't mind if you stare. It's a proud moment for him. See that spark in his eye. Perry saw it when he took the picture in early April 1971. It was Monk's first time back at Snow Ridge in two years. He had just returned from Europe after racing with the U.S. Ski Team. A month earlier he had signed autographs for the Norwegian children. In January he had finished second in the U.S. Ski Association 30-kilometer Championships. His dream of making the Olympics was stronger than ever. Being a U.S. Ski Team member was Monk's answer to his insecurities. He often refers to that accomplishment by saying, "Point proven." Behind Monk is the base lodge of his second home as a kid. He's facing the mountain that now seemed like the 500-foot hill it was. See how proud he is of those brand new Norwegian cross-country racing skies. He skied downhill on them all day.

And no one else there that day wore the U.S. national team suit. If you mention it, he'll go into his closest and bring out his 1969 U.S. Team jacket, which is blue on the outside and red on the inside with a U.S. Ski Team patch like the one in the photo. He'll tell you how the jacket was made in Norway by a manufacturer called Odlo. Then he'll look back at that photo. "I was a stud," he says. "I was king."

Two months later, he had pain in his right knee; he had surgery on it in preparation for the upcoming Olympic try-outs. As serious as the Olympics was to Monk, he didn't let it take away any other fun. Despite his hurt knee, he continued to play intramural softball. He had his surgery postponed two weeks because he skinned his right knee in an intramural soft-ball game. After the surgery he had confidence based on his efforts of his unsuccessful 1968 Olympic tryout, his national team experience and most importantly, his intense training and preparation. But while many of his peers say nobody worked harder, his knee was sore and led to a disappointing performance in tryouts.

That disappointment didn't hinder his pursuit for athletic greatness. Instead of sulking, he started training on a bike. Monk had the cardiovascular and leg strength to compete in a sport like bicycle racing, where there wasn't much strain on his knees. Two U.S. cross-country skiers, Bob Gray and Mike Gallagher, rode competitively in the off-season. In the sum-mer after the 1972 Sapporo Olympics, Monk finished second in the Eastern Bicycle Time-Trial Championships near Kill-ington, Vt. Cross-country didn't work, but maybe I can make the Olympics on a bicycle, he thought. On second thought, he couldn't leave skiing. It was in his blood. Plus, he hated riding in packs and being elbowed, and the thought of possibly crashing onto pavement made skiing even more enticing. He knew he'd never make the Olympics as a skier with his bum knee. So he went the only other route, following in the footsteps of Merrill and taking as Monk says, the "backdoor in" as a coach of the U.S. Ski Team.

Monk began as the U.S. Ski Team Nordic program coordinator, based out of its Denver office, and coached the U.S. Ski Team junior cross-country skiers, which brings us to the next photo above his computer, second from the right. Jim Balfanz, the U.S. Nordic program director at the time, shot that color photo in February 1973 in Leningrad. A couple months earlier Monk had trained the U.S. junior Nordic-combined team in St. Moritz, Switzerland, and had spent his Christmas holiday there and missed his family. His ski friends became his new family. In that photo Monk and the U.S. junior Nordic team are in front of the Bronze Horseman, a famous monument in Senatskaya Square, next to St. Isaac's Cathedral. The statue is on a massive, single piece of red granite and is supposed to be the shape of a cliff. The statue on top is Peter the Great on his horse trampling a snake. The ominous monument is appropriate for the teams competing in the European junior championships in the Soviet Union. The U.S. skiers were the first in the Soviet Union, and they had finished fourth in the boy's 3 x10 km. relay, beating the Norwegians and Swedes. He remembers soldiers holding machine guns in the airport. "The whole country was very intimidating," he says. That winter the U.S. team traveled from Stockholm to

Moscow to Leningrad to Finland to Norway, flying in a small plane with small windows in the Soviet Union. Monk wasn't the only one intimidated that week in Leningrad. All the teams—Finland, France, Poland, Sweden and the United States—applauded when they took off from the airport. In a postcard he sent to his parents, Monk wrote, "Well, I made it out of the USSR alive—so glad to be out of there! (glad to have been too but note the past tense)."

In the fall of 1972, Marty Hall became the first full-time U.S. cross-country team coach. Hall had first met Monk on the Eastern Amateur Ski Association circuit. As the head coach, Hall hired Monk as his assistant before the 1973 fall training. Monk helped organize training camp in Colorado. Then Monk and Marty traveled around Europe with the team that winter.

See how happy Monk is in that color photo to the right of the others? It was taken the morning of the 1973 national cross-country championships in Minneapolis, Minn. He is holding Martha Rockwell's skis in his right arm and smiling at her. He has good reason to smile. Rockwell won every U.S. cross-country skiing championship from 1969 to 1975. "She was the U.S. program," Monk says. On his other side is Hall, who is facing Rockwell. They are standing in the parking lot near Bush Hill on a sunny day. The lack of snow, as seen by the dirt and bare blacktop, didn't seem to bother Martha or Monk.

His absence from law school didn't bother him either. Monk finished his final two terms at Yale in the second semester of 1973 and 1974. Waxing skis and organizing cross-country trails took priority over law textbooks. As he says, he was "playing with the Gods." He'd show up for a week of classes in January and tell his professors, "I'll see you in April." Some of his classmates thought he had dropped out. Then he'd arrive in early April and cram for exams in mid-May. Most students would freak out trying to cover such a voluminous amount of material in a short time span. Not Monk, who never seemed to let on to his friends how much work or stress he faced. He says he never was serious about school, but that he loved challenges, even with his brain. "I gave it my best shot," he says. "I knew I was smart…no big deal." Besides, he knew that if the "piss ants" could pass, he could too. He used four different colored markers to highlight his textbooks. Each color represented a certain level of importance to him so that he prioritized his studying. Looking back, Monk says he wasted his education at Yale because he didn't have time to truly learn the law by discussing and debating with other students. Instead, he filled his mind up like a "bathtub" with information for exams. Of course, he found it more interesting to educate himself about cross-country skiing and training. His experience motivated him to push for a separation between athletics and academics in America, as well as greater funding for amateur international sports such as cross-country skiing.

In the spring of 1974, Monk wrote a 43-page critique, *How the American Can Make It in International Sport: The Case of the Cross-Country Skier*, in his Sociology of Sport class. Law students were allowed to take one undergraduate course per year; Monk chose that class for obvious reasons. In his paper he stated that cross-country is limited to three areas of America: Alaska, Colorado, and Northern New England. And although the U.S. had improved in international competition, its popularity and support couldn't compare with Scandinavian and Central and Eastern European countries. "There are over 280 kilometers of regularly maintained cross-country trails within 15 kilometers of the center of downtown Oslo, Norway, 70 kilometers of which are lighted nightly so that working people can still have a chance to ski everyday," wrote Monk. "Tom Seaver, Joe Namath, and Walter Frazier are each paid at least $100,000 a year (1974 prices) to exhibit their prowess and help New York beat cities like Chicago, but we send teams to international competitions without even a guarantee they will have enough money to get back."

How could the United States compete internationally? Small towns such as Putney, Vt., produced some of the nation's top cross-country skiers.

"It's almost inconceivable that there are four people from a tiny place like Putney, Vermont on the national team," Monk told the *Yale Daily News* in an April 5, 1974 article. "If skiing had been important where John Havlicek grew up, he would have been a great cross-country skier."

After graduating from Yale, he was excited about improving cross-country skiing in America as a coach.

"I'm a total rookie as a coach and snuck right in at the top," Monk told the *Yale Daily News* in an April 5, 1974 article. "But I had a good grasp of the technical aspects and more important—I'm a great waxer."

Monk had become a great waxer after spending countless hours observing his old mentor Merrill. His enthusiasm for his skiers to perform well mirrored his ambitions for himself as a skier. In the fall of 1974, Monk called Cliff Coker, the national head of *Universal* weight machines, and talked him into installing new weights free of charge in the Dartmouth ski team room in Robinson Hall, the same place as the Dartmouth radio station and the school newspaper *The Dartmouth*. This way skiers could lift away from "the football players and Neanderthals around the College gym's weight room."

He also had learned the value of preparation from Merrill. At the time, European teams began training three weeks before the Americans. Monk and Hall decided on a change. As Hall's assistant, Monk searched for a good training camp location, starting in early November, as the Europeans were doing. Monk found a spot in a small snowmobile town a few miles northeast of Yellowstone called Cooke City, Mont.

That brings us to the colored photo right of the Holmenkollen shots. On a sunny November day in 1974, Don Nielsen, a U.S. Ski Team member, took that closeup of Monk with his curly, shaggy brown hair. Looking at it now, Monk says, "I needed a haircut." He didn't need much else, as he refers to that photo day with Monk's Bunch as one of the happiest days of his life. Monk's Bunch, that's what those 13 U.S. Team skiers training in Cooke City with Monk called themselves. At that time, the top two male and two female U.S. cross-country skiers trained with Hall in northern Sweden before going to races in Central Europe. Back in Cooke City, the rest of the elite U.S. skiers stayed in the only inn in town. Cooke City had a population of 40 with no regular grocery store, and mail was delivered only three times a week. But it was cross-country skier heaven. Monk rose early each morning to set tracks in the snow for the team to train. Monk's Bunch also had time to enjoy the jutting mountain peaks, and the old cabins in the middle of nowhere left from miners generations earlier. The team's personality reflected its coach. Driving with the team, Monk played his favorite rock n' roll tapes.

On Monk's shelf above his dry bar he has another picture of that photo day in downtown Cooke City. They were never short on jokes as you can see Monk laughing with Randy Kerr and Ronny Yeager. Monk has yet another picture on his wall, near his window, of his time in Cooke City. That picture is a group shot of the entire team and is framed. Below it is a copy of the inscription inside a book, titled *Rock Dreams*, which the team had given him, and reads: "To MONK, the biggest rocker and roller of them all…THANKS from MONK'S BUNCH for the WINTER of '75."

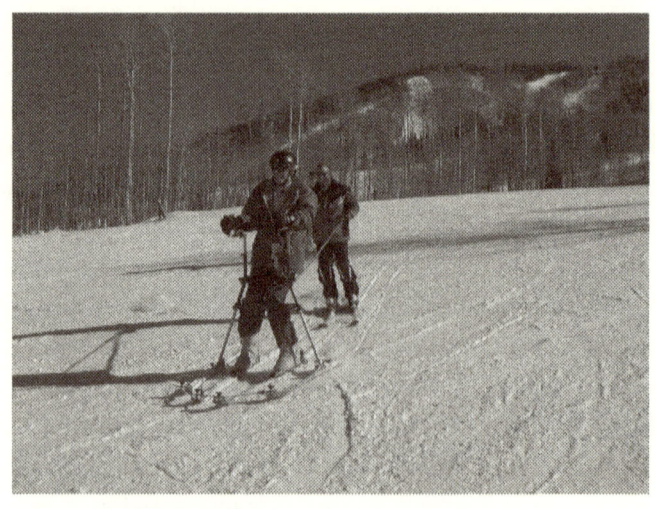

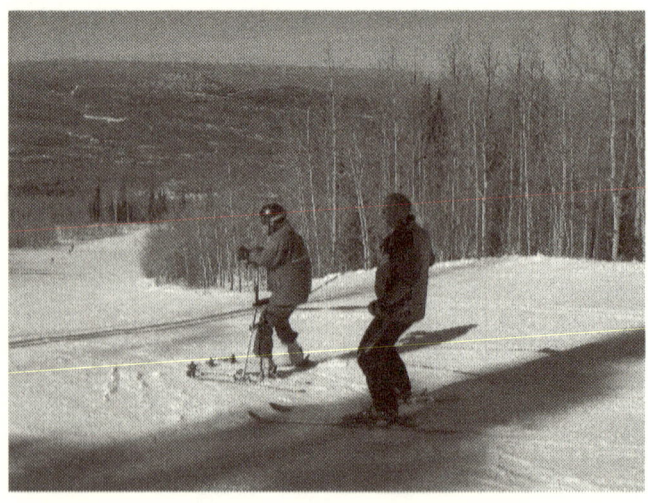

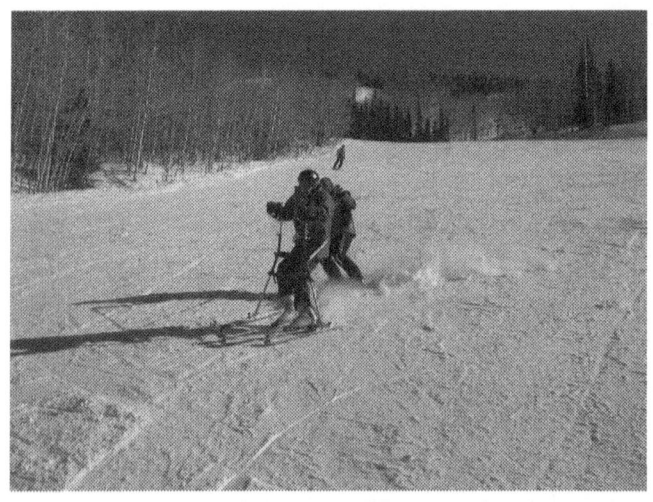

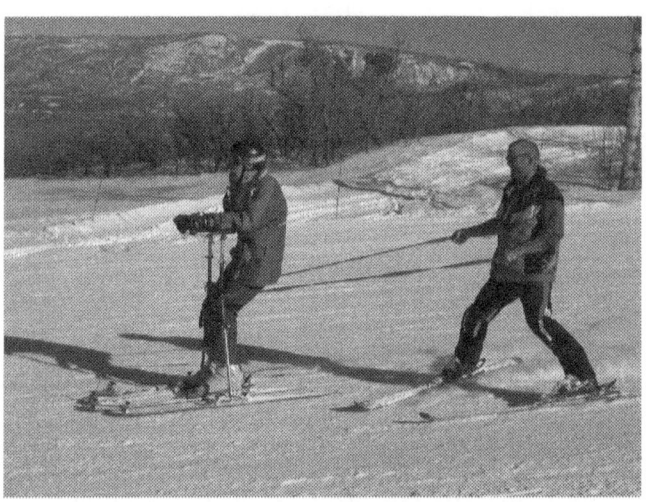

In America, cross-country skiing reached its peak in popularity in the mid-1970s. Not only were more people skiing for recreation, but the Nordic team became more competitive internationally. In 1976 Bill Koch became the first American to medal in cross-country skiing at the Olympics, winning a silver. And Hanover, N.H., was a hotbed for the surging sport. Four Dartmouth skiers were members of the national team: Tim Caldwell; Chris Nice; Don Nielsen; and Douglas Peterson. Caldwell was exceptional. He and Koch were the best in the nation so Hall spent more time with them while Monk spent more time with the other top skiers.

But just when cross-country started becoming popular in America, in large part because of skiers like Monk whose lives were consumed by the sport, he was released as a coach. It was out of his control. He never complained or acted sorry for himself though it was difficult to accept....

John Bower had won the Holmenkollen Nordic-combined race in Oslo, Norway in 1968, which in a non-Olympic or world championship year is equivalent to being the best in the world. Before the 1976 Winter Olympics in Innsbruck, Austria, several changes were made within the U.S. Ski Team. Bower became Nordic program director. He called Monk in the summer of 1975 and told him he had made a coaching change. Bower had hired Tom Upham to replace Monk. Bower and Upham had grown up together in Auburn, Maine.

It's no secret how a man who "lived and breathed" cross-country skiing would feel if his coaching position was taken away. And Monk, at least at first, had that feeling in August 1975. In Hanover, Chris Nice remembers seeing Monk soon after he received word of his dismissal. "He just looked like he had been run over by a truck," says Nice, U.S. Ski Team, 1973-76. "And he should have felt that way because it was totally unfair from our standpoint. He loved the sport with a passion. He gave everything to it and did a super job.... I found Monk had a lot more to offer than Tom."

Monk says he grew more disappointed over his dismissal when he found out Upham, a married man, was having an affair with a female U.S. skier, also married, while *the other female skiers were just pushed aside; hell, ignored.*

To this day Monk doesn't know for sure why Bower fired him, but there are some clues. Nearly a year earlier Monk had taken the cross-country team and trained in Bretton Woods, N.H., because the snow there was better than in Lake Placid, where U.S. officials wanted him to train. That decision created some friction. At the time, Dartmouth and Middlebury had an intense rivalry. So intense that when Monk was in college, Dartmouth coach Al Merrill and Middlebury cross-country coach Bobo Sheehan didn't talk to each other during the season. Bower was from Middlebury, and Monk, obviously a Dartmouth grad.

Monk didn't let anger toward Bower stop him from being involved with the national cross-country scene. He found his next best alternative to coaching, working as a product manager for Trak Skis, the largest cross-country company in the United States. Even though Bower didn't want Monk working for the ski company that was an "official supplier" for the U.S. Ski Team, Monk didn't let it bother him. He still traveled around the world and had fun with his group of ski friends.

In late March 1977, a few weeks before a ski trade show in Las Vegas, Monk noticed his left foot dragging. He didn't pay any attention to it. Then at the trade show, as a representative for Trak Skis, he noticed his left leg involuntarily drag. His left hand clenched up for no reason. The president of Trak Skis told Monk to go to Boston even though he wanted to finish the trade show.

Heading to Brigham & Women's Hospital in Boston on April 10, 1977, Monk's left hand involuntarily clenched up. After a few tests, the doctor told him the news.... Monk had multiple sclerosis. Multiple sclerosis (MS) is as unpredictable as Monk's life has been. There is no proven cause or cure. It is also unknown if a person's condition will improve or worsen. In the United States, about one in a thousand people has MS, according to researchers. Those afflicted, like Monk, have a loss of myelin, which acts as a protective cover for the body's nerve fibers. This affects nerve signals from the brain and damages the central nervous system causing a variety of symptoms, such as numbness, fatigue and trouble walking.

But at the time Monk didn't know what MS was so he didn't worry. Besides, he felt fine and exercised regularly.

In the summer of 1978, he left Trak Skis to put his Yale degree to use, becoming a tax lawyer for a small firm in Laconia, N.H. Monk hated his job. Perry had been pressuring Monk to become a lawyer, preferably in Boonville with him. Monk chose to leave Trak Skis to satisfy his old man. He asked the head of Trak Skis to take him back, but the head of the company wouldn't. The head of Trak Skis felt Monk wasn't as emotionally stable and hungry as he had been, and had chosen to leave the company.

The next two years were the toughest of his life. Skiing was his life, and he had trained and befriended the best in the nation. Now it was gone for a couple reasons beyond his control. First a bum knee, then politics. Now pressure from Perry, and MS. He figured he could still have a "place to play" in Laconia. Most days after work at the law firm, Monk ran at least five miles. On weekends he hiked up New Hampshire mountains, such as Dartmouth's Mount Moosilauke. (The conventional wisdom of the day advised people with MS to "take it easy" and not workout, a scientific belief that has been proven wrong in large part by former Olympic, alpine medalist Jimmie Heuga.) When Monk exercised, he spaced out and didn't concentrate on anything. But no matter how far he ran or how high he climbed he couldn't escape reality. By then most of his Dartmouth and ski friends had moved or were involved in their careers or families. Monk was lonely and scared of his unpredictable disease, but he never told anyone. Although outgoing and likeable, Monk rarely shared his tough and personal issues with friends or family. Cross-country skiers don't complain; they put their heads down and "hammer."

That's why in the fall of 1980 he enrolled at New York University in pursuit of his L.L.M. in tax law. An L.L.M. is a graduate degree in law. He may not have been fond of the law, but he still could be one of the best. In The Dakota he lived with two Yale friends in a second-floor penthouse, owned by the wife of one of his buddies. Monk could barbeque on The

Dakota roof and watch people and taxis zoom in and out of the West 72nd Street entrance to Central Park. His body had different plans. His left leg kept dragging and he felt pins and needles from head to toe when his MS flared up, forcing him to leave after six weeks. By then Perry was putting a load of pressure on Monk to join his Boonville law firm. That pressure caused Monk's relationship with Perry to decline. So Monk turned to his brother and moved in briefly with Dick and his then-wife Georgia in Wolfeboro, N.H.

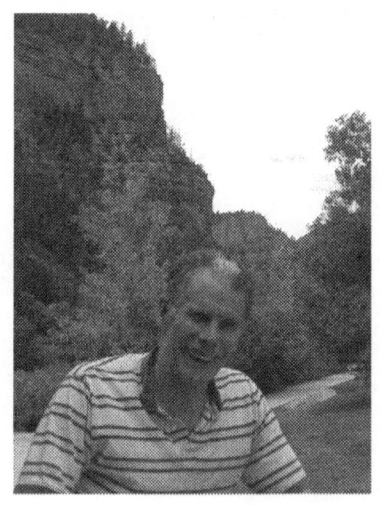

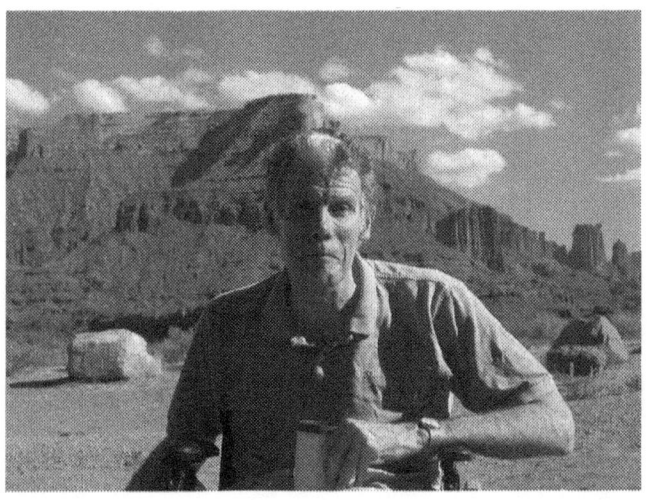

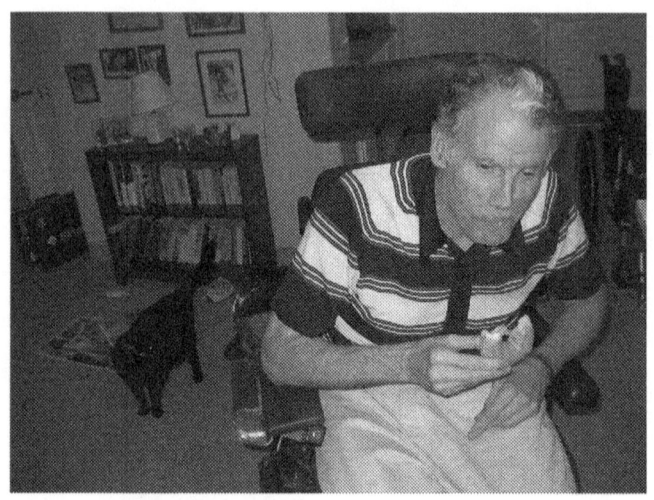

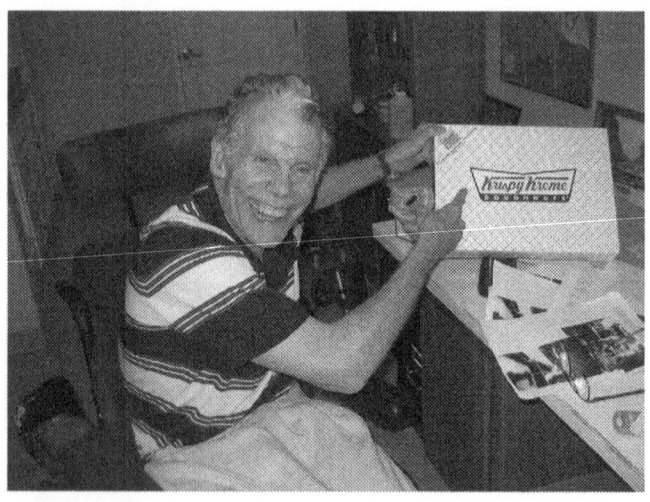

Just after the 1980 Olympics in Lake Placid, John McNamara, a classmate at Deerfield and Dartmouth, set Monk up on a blind date with a friend of his wife's at their house in Rehoboth, Mass. Though Monk had attended two of the most prestigious colleges in America, Dartmouth and Yale, Chris was the brightest girl he had met. Monk's mother was also impressed, telling her, "You're the first woman that's smart enough for Steve."

And their upbeat personalities matched as well. Many of Chris's friends didn't know about her brutal upbringing. But she told Monk how her parents had met at Greenwich High School in Connecticut. She told him how her father had come from Norway and how her mother fell in love with the new foreigner. She told him how he had enlisted as a marine in World War II as well as the Korean War. She told him how her parents were alcoholics and how her father was abusive. She told him how she did everything she could to protect her five siblings. She told him how as the oldest daughter, she tried to fill in as a normal mother to no avail. She told him about her father's physical abuse, similar to marine torture. How he once put a gun to her head and made her pay for the doctor's bill after he broke her jaw. And how he stuffed her head in the toilet and flushed. And how he threw the Christmas dinner against the wall. Then there was the daily stuff. The chronic back pain from him karate chopping her. The loneliness from never being allowed to bring friends, let alone dates, to her home. How could she? Her father might have one of his typical alcoholic tantrums or be passed out in the front yard.

She told him about her mother. How she had upper-class English roots and was more concerned with her status than watching six children. "Don't ever call me mom," she told them. And the initial attraction to the good-looking and intelligent Norwegian she had met in high school had worn away for Chris's mother. In fact, both parents slept in separate bedrooms, each with their own lock and key. It's amazing Chris was able to study with such a broken home. But her parents did give her one good thing: intelligence. She graduated Phi Beta Kappa from Marymount College in Arlington, Va. When she finally did leave her Greenwich home for good, her mother chased her down the driveway with a knife. She never talked to either parent again, and only saw one of her siblings, her older brother Eric, once. Her siblings have since denied any wrongdoing by their parents. Monk never met her family.

Chris showed me how important [and tuff] it is to look forward and live right past and over bad, shabby experiences while still retaining her core essence, her sweetness and caring concern for others.

They lived together in Massachusetts for more than two years. Then they moved to Alexandria, Va., in 1983 and got married. Monk's classmate at Yale Law School, Steve Daniels, lived in Washington, D.C., at the time. Living nearby, Chris babysat for the Daniels family, especially in an urgent circumstance, such as when both parents needed to work while one of their children was sick at home. The Daniels children, like other children, adored Chris. "They liked her so much they almost wanted to get sick," says Steve Daniels.

Chris always wanted to have children of her own and give them a happy childhood she never had. Unfortunately she was unable to have children, a biological problem that tore her apart for the rest of her life.

So she had cats instead. When Monk met her, she owned a 48-pound black cat named Smoke (nicknamed "Tubby" by Monk), whose genetics was the reason for being so fat. She sometimes dressed Tubby in a shirt and pants. Tubby died of a heart attack at age 5. Monk's love for cats developed through Chris, a love that he didn't know then would be more important in his future.

Just after Tubby's death, in the spring of 1983, Monk moved to Washington, D.C. He'd work down there for a few months and then he and Chris would get married and live together. Before he could find a house in Alexandria, Monk stayed with the Daniels. Monk planned to stay a couple weeks until he found a permanent residence. However, just after arriving, he had a MS attack. Unable to get out of bed on his worst days and hobbling up and down the stairs to his third-floor bedroom on his good days, Monk lived with the Daniels for two months or so.

Now look at his wall above his computer. See the plaque. It is left of the six photos. The Democratic staff director gave Monk that brown, wooden plaque with the golden plate and black lettering on June 30, 1987 for his work with the U.S. Senate Committee on Small Business. After leaving the Daniels's house, Monk began working with Sen. Lowell Weicker. Growing up, Chris babysat for Weicker's children in Greenwich, Conn., and later arranged Monk and Weicker to meet. Through that connection, Monk worked for Weicker, then chairman for the U.S. Senate's Committee on Small Business. And Monk received the plaque for his professional competence despite his worsening coordination and speech.

His success in Washington was not enough to keep him there. Monk's roots were in the Northeast. In 1989 he returned to New Hampshire, this time working for one of the three largest law firms in Manchester.

At that time in his life Monk faced many challenges, which he rarely shared with anyone. Monk had trouble speaking clearly and his relationship with Perry worsened. Ruth had died in the spring of 1986 and Perry remarried a woman from Maine a year and a half later. Years earlier, when Monk was at Yale, Perry had promised him, with Ruth present, that he'd stop putting pressure on his son to work for his law firm. After Ruth's death, Perry tried pressuring Monk again. Chris called Perry "The Bull." To Perry, having his youngest son nearby and practicing law together seemed like a great idea. But Monk had seen the world. He couldn't return to the "sticks" of New York. In the winter of 1991 Perry had a stroke and was in a Boonville nursing home for three years. He asked Chris, never Monk, to take him out of the nursing home and drive him home. Perry died in 1995. He left a bequest to the National MS Society, the only sign of sympathy he ever showed toward Monk's disease.

Monk's struggles with MS also worsened. His speech problem had come to the point where he rarely picked up a telephone. When he crossed the street during his lunch break, Ed Damon, a fraternity brother who captained the Dartmouth ski team and was named the best 4-event skier in the country in 1969, remembers it taking him two full lights to walk across on his forearm crutches. Traffic would back up as Monk shuffled back to work.

Many skiers who had lost touch were surprised to see Monk walking on crutches into Al Merrill's funeral. Monk had mentioned to Chris so many tales about Merrill over the years that she once said, "He was at least the second most important male in my life." Merrill died in 1990 and a generation of cross-country skiers attended his funeral in Lebanon, N.H. Monk ignored John Bower and Tom Upham. The others he enjoyed seeing. Randy Kerr thanked him for standing up for him at the 1974 Norwegian Ski Games or Holmenkollen. That year, Monk's Bunch had been in a series of races in Sweden. After the races Monk met Marty Hall in Norway for Holmenkollen. Hall had said before going to Europe that the top U.S. racer in Sweden could race in Norway. Kerr was the top racer, but Hall had second thoughts about him going to Holmenkollen. Monk helped convince Hall that Kerr should go. At Merrill's funeral Monk told Kerr, "You deserved it. You deserved it."

As the years passed Monk's MS symptoms affected his job and home life. In 1993, the Manchester law firm released Monk because of his difficultly communicating with other lawyers. By that time he didn't have much interest in his job as tax lawyer and retirement planner. He always liked people; not the law. Plus, he received a good disability retirement package. His speech problem carried over to his personal life. Often Chris translated phone calls and conversations with friends.

The speech isolated him more and more over the years. Everything but his mind declined. In 1993 he put on cross-country skis for the last time of "true stride and glide."

Work and skiing were gone but he still had Chris. Without being able to have her own children, her heart was broken. Her spirit wasn't. She made it her life's duty to help Monk, such as answering his phone calls. "She was the most positive person I ever met," he says.

A few years after his retirement, Monk received a phone call from his Dartmouth fraternity brother, Buzz Land, who was on his way from Vermont to Cape Cod with his wife Donna for the weekend. Because of a March snowstorm on route, Buzz pulled off an exit in Manchester and decided to call Monk. He hadn't seen Monk in many years. He couldn't understand him on the phone so Buzz told Monk he'd wait at a Burger King in Manchester. About a half hour or so later Monk arrived by himself. Buzz and Donna noticed his feet dragging. They also noticed his huge smile, and a twinkle in his eye similar to the expression in his photos. They reminisced and laughed about their college years for a couple hours. Then they hugged and Monk walked with his forearm crutches to the handicap ramp.

"Monk, let me give you a hand," said Buzz.

Monk looked at him.

"You're not going to let me help you, are you?"

Monk just smiled, and then slalomed down the icy ramp, using his crutches like ski poles. After Monk drove away Buzz cried, and as he turned onto the highway, he thought to himself, "If I ever hear one of my kids complain or if I ever complain again, then shoot me. Because he just has zero to complain about what is going on for his life."

Years later Buzz invited Monk to meet for lunch at the Hanover Inn restaurant. Buzz waited. No Monk. He waited. Still no Monk. Finally, he walked out of the restaurant and onto the street. There was Monk, alone on his crutches trying to fix his flat tire, having never asked for help.

Each of Monk's old college or ski friends seem to have similar reactions upon visiting him after years of separation. For instance, John Morton reunited with Monk in 1997, and several days afterward said in a commentary for Vermont Public Radio: "We suffered through some grueling competitions together in college; demanding race courses, freezing temperatures, and difficult snow conditions. But nothing we faced as Nordic skiers compares with the challenges my old buddy confronts now, each day, with grit and a remarkable sense of humor." What his friends continue to marvel at is how his sense of humor hasn't changed, despite everything he has faced.

He had been enduring the battle with MS, but soon that wouldn't be his toughest challenge. On St. Patrick's Day in 1998, life seemed somewhat normal. He felt fine, no major MS symptoms. Chris was in her usual positive spirit. Everything next happened so fast. Two weeks later, on a Sunday, Chris felt weak. She asked Monk to drive her two miles from their home to Elliot Hospital in Manchester. He dropped her off, and returned home and ate dinner. After he finished, the phone rang. The doctor told him that Chris was going to die soon of kidney and liver failure—maybe less than a day, maybe weeks, but soon. After he hung up the phone, Monk sped to the hospital with uncertain thoughts on his mind: She might not make it through the night…. How will she be when I get to the hospital?

Chris talked and laughed with him and her roommate. Monk didn't believe a word the doctor said. She'd make it. He was sure of it. And she herself had never mentioned that the doctors had told her she was going to die. He was so sure that he signed a contract a week later to buy a new house for them.

How quickly life can change. Monk had learned that from a knee injury and from John Bower and from MS. But Chris too? No, God couldn't be so cruel…. Four weeks after the diagnosis Monk gave Chris a big goodbye hug. "Make her as comfortable as you can for as long as you can," Monk told the doctor just after their final embrace. "I knew it was our last conscious time," he says, putting his fingers through each other…. The next day she lost consciousness.

On the evening of May 5, 1998, Chris died in her sleep. In Monk's letter to Chris's friends, he wrote:

….Chris accepted with never a complaint whatever life did or didn't give to her, as well as all the limitations and extra physical and emotional strains for her my MS brought. She was my true love, life partner, best friend, and my legs and oral contact with the outside world, as well as my constant emotional leaning post….

For Monk, losing Chris was the worst thing he ever faced. Sure he had his tragic moments involving skiing and MS. This was different. Any other person would have fallen like a beginning skier on a double diamond. So maybe this is the point where he crumbles and goes into a depression and feels sorry for himself.... Not Monk. Not a man who hasn't cried like a baby since 1965 for a reason which he has since forgotten. Not for a man who expended so much effort that he had spit hanging down to his waist after ski races. Instead, Monk decided to do what he's always done when facing something uncomfortable, he simply put his head down and "hammered."

"He has a spirit that is as broad as all outdoors and is as deep as the ocean," says Carroll Brewster. "The guy is a very deeply driven kind of person of great goodness and deep perception of other people and huge passion. When you put all those together, I think you can stand up to most everything that's thrown at you and he has."

For the next two months Monk lived by himself in Manchester. He wasn't the only one deeply affected by Chris's death. Two months later, her cat Angel also died. Monk's four cousins, who lived in Hartford, Conn., left him prepared meals to heat. He spent time visualizing life without Chris and thought how he would communicate with his friends and what activities he could do.

Cooking and cleaning and daily living became too much of a burden. And hobbling around on forearm crutches didn't make it any easier. Monk's cousins still helped him, but they had families of their own to help. Two months after Chris's death, Monk moved to The Gables, an assisted living complex in Farmington, Conn.

White heads and dead heads. That's what Monk, at 52 years old the youngest resident by a long shot, jokingly called his neighbors living at The Gables. For his next five years it was a lonely place. He went from using forearm crutches to a wheelchair. Monk thought the residents and workers were too formal and not very friendly. Only dinner was served, which he ate at the cafeteria. He had to buy groceries and make breakfast and lunches, or as he liked to then, eat fast food. Monk had to pay for every service. He remembers falling out of his wheelchair and being charged for help back up on it.

He did have some old college and ski friends visit. But his visitors only stayed a few hours and then he was alone again. Even his brother couldn't stay too long because he sold liability insurance to ski areas across the nation.

Now we're back to those skiing photos. He hung them on his walls and placed them on his shelves to keep himself from going crazy. One time when Brewster visited Monk, he looked at Monk's collection of skiing medals and patches and ribbons in his glass display case. Then he turned his head and looked at Monk, who without pity or angst, said, "Stud turned dud."

His friends' views of him hadn't changed. Not too many people in wheelchairs drive themselves to go lift weights and use the treadmill three days a week, as Monk did in his Subaru wagon. He'd hoist his wheelchair into the trunk of his car and then drive off.

Besides working out at the gym, he spent most of his time in his room, making meals or on the Internet. For Monk, the Internet was a rose in the middle of a thornbush. Without e-mail, he had no contact with the outside world. His speech problem had come to the point where he could order a pepperoni pizza with extra cheese or communicate in a yes-no telephone conversation, but not much else. That had been Chris's job.

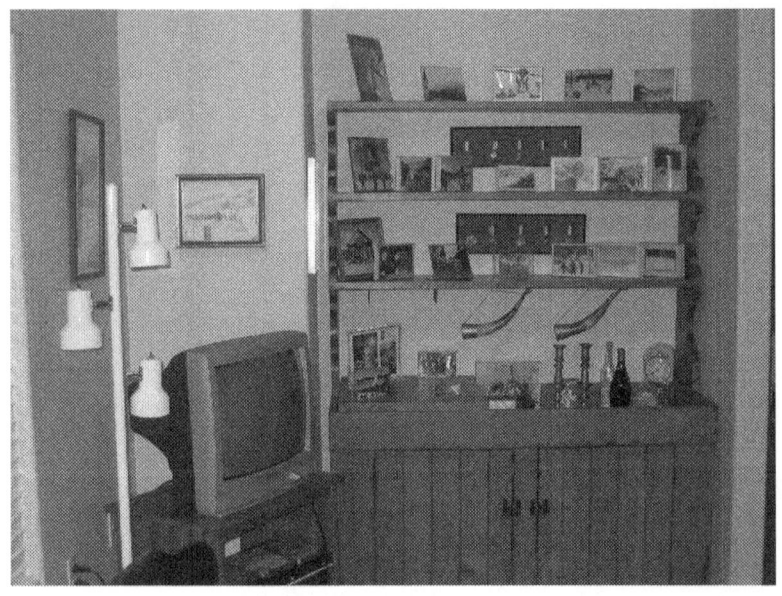

His speech problem became the most difficult MS setback for him to accept. Monk's life became lonelier. He grew more distant from his cousins as they became more involved in their own lives. He corresponded online with a lady in Hartford, but after a while he realized it wouldn't turn into anything more than that. His only physical activity involved lifting weights and using the treadmill three days a week. To make matters worse, he had nowhere to go. His brother lived in Arizona and heat was bad for MS. Besides, he had lived in the East his entire life and had many of his friends there. His medical contacts were in Boston.

In March 2003, Dick moved to Grand Junction, Colo., and was retired. That is when Monk began talking to him about a change. But he had never been to Grand Junction, at least not since his competitive skiing days and that was just driving by. He had never seen the assisted living home he might live in. He still viewed his brother like an uncle and hadn't lived close by since they were kids. He didn't know any doctors in Grand Junction. And he hadn't heard about the various activities they had in the area for disabled people. Yet as Dick says, "It was an incredible leap of faith."

Monk decided he needed an advocate when going to see the doctors. He knew his life with MS couldn't be much worse than where he was. In October 2003, Monk left the East, his roots, and didn't look back, flying to an assisted living home in Grand Junction. Monk's niece, Wendy, who lived a couple hours away in Basalt, Colo., found a ski instructor to drive a U-Haul truck full of Monk's belongings across country. When that truck arrived and turned into the parking lot, a big sign stood there and read:

> The Commons of Hilltop
> …living made easy

Red letters move across his black computer screen: "Bozo and Monk live here." It sounds like an odd mix—a clown and a religious man living together. And it is a weird relationship, but not in the way you think.

One Sunday I was pushing Monk through the main corridor of The Commons when I said, "Did you go to church today?"

"No," he said.

"No, why not?"

"Bozo is my God."

Bozo is Monk's fat black cat. Since Chris's death, Bozo has been Monk's everyday companion.

On his wall near the bathroom, he has a photo of Chris holding a treat for Bozo, who is standing on his hind legs and appears normal size. Bozo has become fatter living with just Monk, who refers to himself as Bozo's dad. Bozo purrs and sometimes drools while Monk snaps his tail "like a towel in a men's locker room." Sometimes he jokes that it is foreplay and that since Bozo was neutered his tail has become his new source of pleasure. Monk started this affectionate antic on Booboo, his previous cat, who liked it so much that he decided to train Bozo as a kitten. Now Bozo can't get enough;

he also enjoys lying on his back with his paws in the air like a dog and having his belly rubbed.

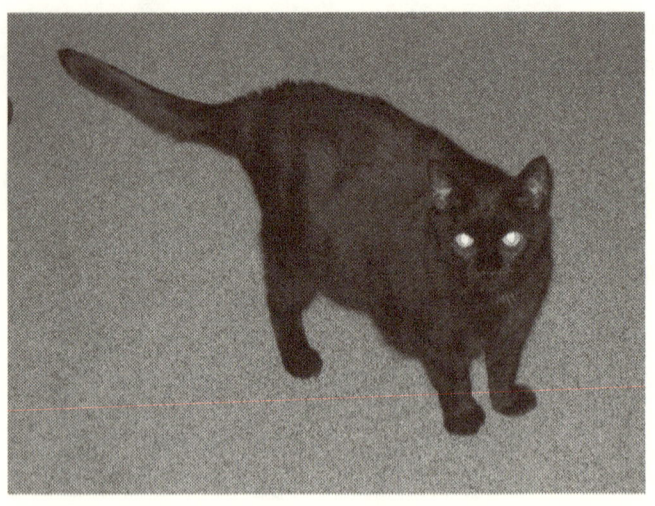

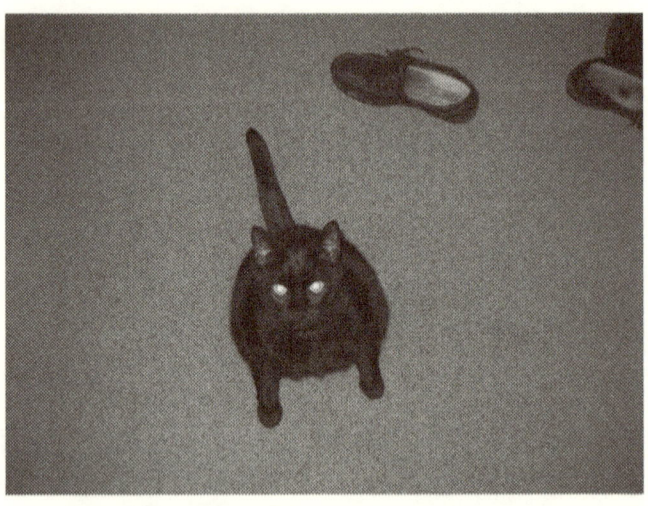

Like Bozo, Monk wants affection, but Monk's speech has isolated him from life outside The Commons.

If there is one positive thing MS has done for Monk, it involves his relationship with Dick. Because of the disease he made the choice to move to Grand Junction, and for the first time since Boonville, live permanently close to his brother. Dick has always been very allergic to cats. Since Monk moved five miles away, Dick visits almost every day and has built up a greater tolerance for Bozo. Dick, like Monk, is a private man, but through the frequent visits he and Monk have become close enough that they both see each other now as brothers instead of uncle and nephew. As kids, Monk had resembled Perry and both were right-handed; Dick had looked like Ruth and both were left-handed. They look more like brothers now, both have tall lanky frames and small waves in their hair, which seem to always stay in place. Some days Dick brings Monk groceries. However, unlike The Gables, Monk eats three meals a day in The Commons' cafeteria. Eating is much more enjoyable than at The Gables as Monk teases and jokes with the wait staff. Monk can be himself.

Moving from The Gables to The Commons, a simple and yet noticeable difference is on his name tag near his door, which now less formally reads: "Steve Williams and Bozo." Inside is the Monk Museum. Covering most of his beige walls, there still are those framed pictures. He keeps other pictures, cross-country stories and documents from his past in the black filing cabinet to the left of his desk. His manual wheelchair rests there, and is folded up. Next to the chair are Bozo's bowls.

His desk is cluttered with documents and e-mails that he's printed out, as well as an occasional empty *Fritos* wrapper or issue of *Adirondack Life* magazine, and a cross-country book or two, items that recollect his past. There may be little point in putting everything in folders or neat piles since Bozo walks onto his desk when he pleases, knocking papers on the floor. Monk doesn't seem to mind, as he says, "It's his house."

On the other side of his desk is a pair of big windows looking out from the second floor onto the parking lot. In front of the windows, there is a glass display case with Monk's medals and patches and ribbons neatly organized, as well as a black Deerfield Academy chair his parents gave him for graduation. There are pictures on each of his shelves above his wooden dry bar, which is across from his computer, on the far side of the room. There are pictures of Chris and Al Merrill and Marty Hall and John Morton and…. On the floor and against the remaining wall space are two wooden bookshelves filled with books primarily about law and politics and skiing and Monk's interests, books such as "Locked In the Cabinet" by Robert B. Reich (he worked as secretary of labor under President Bill Clinton), who Monk remembers as a nice guy who lived three doors down from him in Smith Hall freshman year at Dartmouth, and "All I Need to Know I Learned From My Cat" by Suzy Becker.

His main room is connected to two small bedrooms: one for him and one for Bozo. Above his bed is a framed poster of Holmenkollen, which he calls "the Yankee Stadium of ski areas." A bathroom completes his personal living space at The Commons.

Most days Monk sits in his automatic wheelchair, reading or typing e-mails to his circle of family and friends he refers to as "Monk's Mafia." He types more now than when he practiced law, using his right hand and occasionally pressing the shift key with his left index finger. He wears pants and a short-sleeve collared shirt and brown shoes. He refills his decanter glass, which is always within arm's length. When he leaves his room, he keeps the glass in a black pouch strapped to his wheelchair. When a visitor arrives, he takes off his reading glasses and turns off MSNBC on his television. Then he presses his knob on his wheelchair so he can face the visitor and smiles…. Only if you ask and patiently listen to many garbled phrases he repeats until you understand will you know how he *really* feels.

"I miss the phone," he says. "Thank God for computers. I would be in deep shit. Would I still be funny?"

Maybe not to outsiders, but those in The Commons still would notice his daily antics. Monk takes sleeping pills to go to bed because he has so much energy. He presses the speed-control switch on his wheelchair and zooms down the hallway as if it were the Indianapolis 500. He uses that enthusiasm when he works out as well.

"It's never too early to begin preparing for the demands and arduous rigors of skiing…. if using a treadmill, you can run it as slow as a mere 0.8 miles per hour as you pace away. Don't be bashful; accept realities, and this is said by a former sub 2-minute half-miler in college…. So, being disabled is no excuse to not be as fit as you possibly can be," Monk wrote in the Colorado Discover Ability October 2004 newsletter.

As you know by now, Monk isn't a talker. He's a doer. He hasn't stopped lifting weights since he began at Dartmouth in 1967. That's why every Monday, Wednesday and Friday morning he rides on a bus that takes him and a few old men from The Commons just around the corner to St. Mary's Life Center. He does the same hour and a half exercise routine every time—10 to 15 reps, moving his wheelchair from one machine to the next. He starts with his legs: leg extensions; leg curls; leg presses; gets a drink of water; leg abductors; and adductors. Then he parks his chair in front of one of the 10 treadmills against the wall and facing a row of big windows. Outside it is cloudy. The wind has blown nearly all the leaves from one of the two trees in the grassy courtyard. Monk slowly walks onto the treadmill farthest to the right. He is hunched over at the waist, taking small, laborious steps at 0.8 miles per hour. He's wearing a safety magnet, which is attached to the treadmill and his T-shirt incase he can't keep up, which happens. The magnet unclips and the treadmill stops. He presses a button to slow it down to 0.7 miles per hour. He keeps taking those small steps with his skinny legs as he holds onto the treadmill handrails, staring at the numbers and little dots that blink on the monitor.

A while later he is doing reps on the military press machine. He takes a deep breath after the first set and pats his shoulders and says with a smile, "Wake up boys. Wake up boys." Behind him, there is a white banner that reads:

<u>ST. MARY'S</u>—Because life is what <u>you</u> make it!
LIFE CENTER

Monk's condition hasn't gotten worse since Chris died, and it has even become steadier since moving to Colorado. MS can affect cognitive abilities. In Monk's case, there are two things that his disease has not affected: his mind; and his spirit....

Back in 1999, he had tried skiing alone at Okemo, in Ludlow, Vt. That had been his last time skiing. He fell so many times it took him three hours to complete one run. But in January 2004, just a few months after moving to Grand Junction, he became a stud. Monk skied again. This time was different than at Okemo. Dick and his wife Genie drove Monk through the towering mesa mountains of western Colorado to nearby Powderhorn. Monk joined his niece, Wendy, and her husband at the mountain. Wendy helped arrange Monk with Tyler Jones, an instructor who runs an adaptive ski program at Powderhorn. Noticing Monk's hunched posture and awkwardness standing, both due to MS, Jones hooked him into a "ski slider." In addition to his normal boots and skis, which is a frame built like a walker on skis, Monk rested his forearms on a pair of medal ski crutches or outriggers. So he had four skis or a four-ski frame, all roped together for stability. Jones then skied behind Monk, holding two chords attached to the outriggers to help control Monk's speed, balance and direction. Since that great day Monk e-mails his periodic outdoor activities—many times with flashbacks of his Hanover days or with the national team—to "Monk's Mafia," as he wrote about that first day back on skis:....*Great weather: 35 degrees, sun and soft snow; not to rub it in the noses of you Easterners with your 0 degree temperature and your bullet proof powder, but the West is really the best.*

Thrilled to be back on skis, Monk didn't seem to mind his blunders on the slope. A month after his first trip to Powderhorn, he realized that his weekly trips on the ski slider with Jones's chords don't guarantee a smooth ride. On his second run of his second time out on a steep trail Monk lost his balance and one of Jones's chords broke free. Monk skied in a circle, going uphill, and fell backward. His body and head struck the hard-packed snow and the ski slider fell into his lap. Jones had to readjust the ski slider.

Monk's next trip to Powderhorn, he used a ski slider built for a lighter skier, and suffered three more crashes similar to the original one. Despite Dick skiing backward and holding Monk's ski tips in position as he looked between his legs for other skiers and snowboarders, Monk didn't have much control.

The R side arm rest/handle actually got loose enuff that it would pop up w/ the speed and ease to be expected of a college guy "slugging" beers at his fraternity bar; don't know but at least as I have heard.

With his ski slider, loading onto and off the ski lift is an adventure despite the chairlift attendant slowing it down. The ski slider rests on Monk's lap as he rides up. Jones keeps his ski between Monk's skis for support as he unloads. Monk's last 2004 trip to Powderhorn proved it isn't easy.

I was slow once getting up [standing up] from my chairlift seat and as my ski instructor and I unloaded w/ the ski slider, my R ski got caught in the orange traffic cones the area had on the R edge of the unloading ramp and I pealed off over the edge of the unloading ramp thru untracked snow. Since the instructor puts a ski in w/ my skis as we load and ride the lift uphill, he came along w/ me over the edge in the soft, untracked snow into the puckerbush at the top. So, another compliment to the instructor.

Many former national team skiers, even good non-competitive skiers, would be frustrated in Monk's position. Instead he exudes laughter and thanks to those involved, including The Commons' staff, who prepare his bag lunch for Powderhorn.

Management should appreciate the short, white-haired lady who approached me at dinner, asking how my skiing went today. She left w/ the comment of how lucky I am to have a brother who does so much to see I get to ski. Absolutely; in spades.

The end of ski season didn't end Monk's activities. In May he camped out and went rafting with Jones and a group of disabled people in eastern Utah. They paddled down the Colorado River in inflatable two-person kayaks, resembling canoe-shaped rafts.

The list of first-time-in-a-while activities continued for Monk. In June he rode a bike using hand pedals. He dodged joggers and regular bike riders as he rode on the paved path along the Colorado River in Grand Junction.

By then any apprehension he had before moving to Colorado disappeared when he hit the ski slope. After a summer of rafting and biking, Grand Junction seemed like a good decision, as he concluded his e-mail about the biking trip, *Thanx to all for your interest and encouragement, The Monk is back.* Then again, he signs off under various aliases: *Monk and Bozo; Bozo and dad; Bozo's dad; the Bozo boys; the Bozos; both of the Bozos; Monk's Bozo; meow meow [Bozo's signature, as per his personal secretary Monk]; head Bozo.* He always had a knack for one-liners, even before his speech difficulty.

"He was enormously skilled in the English language," Brewster says. "Every college has its lingo and particularly because Dartmouth is as isolated as it is, it has a very special lingo. And in our time a great deal of it was invented in the imagination of Steve Williams."

"Head Bozo" began the 2005 ski season with Jones and Dick in January. On the drive to Powderhorn in Dick's truck, dark clouds loomed over the mesa mountains, prompting a Monk flashback that in many ways applies to much of his life.

The threat of blowing snow this day reminded me of my 1ˢᵗ XC race for Dartmouth College, the Franconia Nordics, near the base of NH's Cannon Mtn…My legs were chilled right thru the front panels of my knickers, and my wool knicker socks only collected more snow to later melt and chill my legs while dripping moisture from melted snow into my boots. Major chill then but not this past FR. Not a story of success but just survival.

In 2005 Powderhorn had some of the best snowfall in the recent memory of locals. Monk took advantage skiing weekly. Occasionally, when Jones was available, he skied two consecutive days, something he hadn't done since 1993. Reverting back to his fraternity days, he had a few drinks after skiing if time permitted. Malibu Rum, a coconut flavored rum, became his new favorite.

As the season progressed he gained confidence and his legs grew stronger. By chance one day, Monk and Jones skied down Powderhorn's terrain park near the bottom of the mountain. Upon skiing through the park and watching other skiers and snowboarders do jumps and tricks, Monk decided he could too. Sure enough he headed toward a ramp and "caught some air" with his ski slider and chords! Here we are again, the old Monk at Snow Ridge, this time, ski slider and all, a smooth landing. The season continued with runs down the terrain park, "catching air," and warm spring skiing concluded the year.

He rafted down the Colorado River with the same group this spring as last. He didn't stop there, adding waterskiing and yoga to his activity list. On a hot July day he waterskied on Lake Mirage, a long, skinny private lake next to Interstate 70 near Grand Junction. Sitting on a padded seat connected to a metal frame with outriggers and a mono-ski, Monk took three laps around the lake, scooting over big wakes as it conjured up childhood memories of waterskiing in upstate New York. The next day, he skied again at Lake Mirage, this time intending to ski on two regular skis. The instructors were hesitant. Monk talked them into it. After two failed attempts, he rose out of the water, hunchback and all. The people on the boat flashed pictures in amazement as he rode three times, the last across the entire lake.

He seems to get the same reaction wherever he is. After visiting Monk in The Commons two summers ago, Ed Damon was walking down the hallway with his wife when an elderly woman asked whom he had visited. Damon told her, Steve Williams. "I never met him," said the old woman. "But I hear he's a very brilliant man."

Part of the reason elderly people admire him is because he does what most of them can't or won't do, such as eating whatever he wants in large quantities. Calories or cholesterol have never been a major concern for Monk. He's maintained a skinny frame his entire life. In New Haven he often ate lunch at Louis' Lunch, on Crown Street. He'd order a hotdog with bacon wrapped around it, known as "pig in a blanket." Now, Monk loves glazed Krispy Kreme donuts almost as much as Bozo loves having his tail snapped. The fact he drools onto his lap and his fingers are sticky is of little concern. He says he has hollow legs when it comes to eating. I witnessed that one day when I visited him and brought a dozen glazed Krispy Kreme donuts. Two hours later, standing to leave, I asked Monk how long the donuts would last him. He held up his right index finger and smiled and said, "One." He had only one donut left for himself. He had eaten 10 and gave one to me for the road. Vintage Monk.

On my ride home I couldn't help but think about a Peanuts cartoon he had shown me. One morning at breakfast in Norway in March 1973, Marty Hall had handed Monk a cartoon from the *International Herald Tribune*. In the comic strip, Snoopy knocks on the door with his bowl in his mouth, implying he wants food. Charlie Brown answers the door and remarks on how Snoopy's hunger strike didn't last long. "I learned something," said Snoopy. "The brain may be important...but the stomach is still in charge!"

Unfortunately, when he wants to eat out at Taco Bell, which is just over a mile away, he is at the mercy of Dick or a friend for a lift. When offered to take a road trip, possibly to Aspen, Monk wrote to me:

The whiteheads and deadheads I look at daily here at Geriatric Junction [or Menopause Manor] need to be replaced in my scenic radar, please.... all residents at Bozo's bar and grill will be dressed, fed and ready to go by 10, tho he might continue eating after we leave....

Last fall Monk and I went on a couple of road trips. It was the first time he had been farther east of Powderhorn since moving to Grand Junction. I drove over the Colorado River and past the high mesas on both sides of the highway. We traveled past snow-capped Mount Sopris on Highway 82 and along Independence Pass, a narrow, winding mountain road that often is without a rail guard, which scared Monk. He said he was worried about Bozo not having a dad. On the way back to Grand Junction, I saw a car with a John Elway license plate. "People in Colorado love John Elway," I said.

"He's God to them," Monk said.

"I know it. He must be the most famous person in Colorado."

"He shits ice cream."

One day, we drove on Highway 133, past Mount Sopris and onto a dirt road. We came to Beaver Lake, a small body of water that reflected the autumn leaves on the bell-shaped mountain behind it. Monk told me he had to pee. For Monk, even an everyday habit like using the bathroom becomes a task. So I wheeled him over to a small, wooden restroom building with a blue roof and blue doors. Inside the men's door was a green, plastic cylinder, about knee-high, that resembled a toilet without a seat or lid. I helped Monk take short steps to the toilet. He struggled to lift his right pant leg.

Finally, he pulled it up high enough. His drainage bag and spout were hidden as I saw nothing but pee flow out from behind the cuff of his pant leg. He somehow barely missed his pant leg and brown Timberland shoes. Then we both started laughing. I think it was because I told Monk he was nearly peeing on himself. As we laughed, the heel of his shoe got pee on it. This went on for a while. I told him he had a cleaner shoe. Monk struggled to turn off the spout and got a little bit of pee on his hands. As he tried to lift his leg down, it got stuck for a moment on the rim of the bowl. We both laughed again.

That was a good time. But he doesn't go on trips every day. There are many lonely days, even with Dick around. Dick drives him for his monthly catheter change and to the doctor's. Even after lifting weights or going on a skiing or rafting trip, he's back in his room with Bozo, the youngest residents in The Commons. He views his elderly neighbors as acquaintances rather than friends. Just in the last few months, Monk's neighbors, next to him and across the hall, both died. Another man on Monk's floor, who had become paraplegic in a skiing accident over 30 years ago and had written an autobiography, died in July, just two months after his book was published.

So here we are, again, admiring those photos on his wall.

Those photos make Monk more aware of his past, and in a way, optimistic about his future. So in many ways he needed his skiing life and the photos he kept to make the most of his life with MS. "Reminds me of fond memories and I smile. Better than this fucking thing," he says, pointing to his wheelchair. "They remind me of where I was and what I could do and that I'm still the same person, but not quite. I'm the 59-year-old version of that." Then he pauses and smiles and says: "Monk the hunk."

He wants a female companion and to get married, but he says it is like a "Hail Mary pass." But this story can't end on a "desperation heave" considering he's been catching gutsy first-down passes across the middle his entire life.

But the photographs are reminders of his great past. Some left in. Some left out.

On Sept. 17, 2004, I traveled on a bus with Monk and about a dozen other people with some type of handicap to a remote campsite outside of Moab, Utah. Sitting on the bus that was parked in front of The Commons someone asked an Americore volunteer, named Joy, where she was from. "I've lived in Grand Junction my whole life," she said.

"You have more life ahead of you," said Monk.

We arrived in late afternoon, and set up our tents. We had time before dinner and I asked Monk if he wanted to go explore and see the Colorado River, which could be heard nearby. He said, "It's up to you." So I pulled Monk backward in his wheelchair through the sand and soft dirt near our campsite. This way his footrests wouldn't slide into the loose ground. I pulled him along this winding and hilly and some-times bumpy path in order to avoid small trees and brush. We were about 30 feet from the Colorado River, when I asked Monk if he wanted me to pull him close to see it. He said, "It's up to you." I told him it's worth a try, and pulled him down a steep and narrow path to a point where we could go no far-ther. We took some pictures of the desert mesa that towered over the river in front of us. With little room to move because of the thick vegetation, I began to pull Monk back up the path. I pulled and twisted and did whatever I could to get him up this steep incline. We were near the top of the thicket with the steepest part of the path ahead. I pulled as hard as I could, but it was no use. So as he stood up, I lifted the wheelchair and placed it on level surface at the top. Monk was hunched over, barely standing, his knees and skinny legs at an awkward position. I tried to help him by having him put his left arm around my neck and shoulders. It was no use. Monk told me to switch to the other arm, which I did on his right side. We both were struggling, stuck in this spot just a few feet away from his wheelchair and no one within shouting distance. This went on for a while, with Monk trying to walk up and me using all my energy to make sure he didn't fall. It came to a point where I thought it might be appropriate for Monk to blurt some four-letter words as to question my reasoning and judgement for allowing him to be in this predicament. But, at that point, he started…laughing, and saying something which I couldn't understand. So I started laughing. There we were, Monk with his arm around me jabbering undecipherable words and laughing, and me laughing so hard I almost let him go and fall down. That's when I understood what "Monk's Mafia" meant. No photos needed.

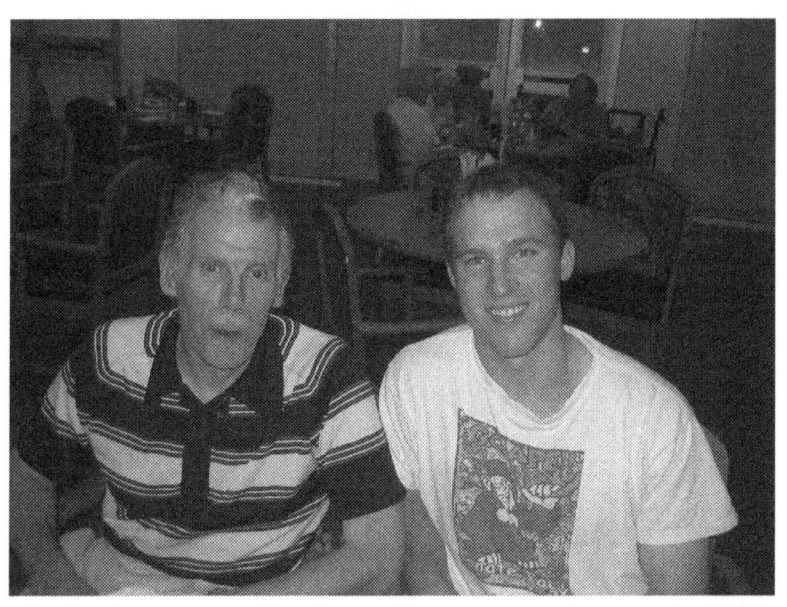

The Monk and the author at The Commons.

978-0-595-38626-0
0-595-38626-1